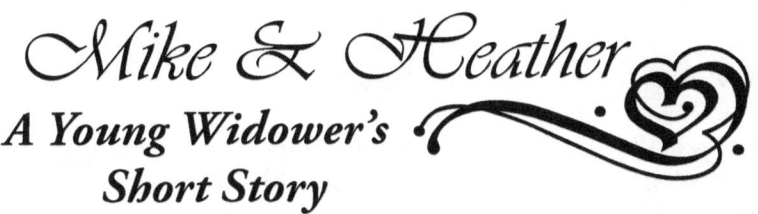

Mike & Heather
A Young Widower's
Short Story

Michael E. Cohen

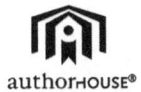

authorHOUSE®

AuthorHouse™
1663 Liberty Drive
Bloomington, IN 47403
www.authorhouse.com
Phone: 1-800-839-8640

First published by AuthorHouse 6/5/2009

ISBN: 978-1-4389-8197-0 (sc)
ISBN: 978-1-4389-8198-7 (eb)

Printed in the United States of America
Bloomington, Indiana

This book is printed on acid-free paper.

Dedication

This book is dedicated to my late wife Heather, my parents, the McCarthy family, the new people in my life that I love, and all the people who help me continue on my journey in this world. And to all the people who have lost a loved one to cancer.

I'd also like to mention my friends Steven, Diego, and sister-in-law's husband Gary, for their indispensable help in the computer area that I know nothing about. With out them, I would have not gotten this book written. I also would have shot my computer with my 12 Gage!

Contents

Introduction

I wanted to write this book mainly for other widow*ers*. This was because when I went looking for books to read on the subject of grief, I found that they where geared more for women then men. The book I finally did read, mentioned widowers, and talked about grief in some general terms, but still gave me the impression that it was for women more than men.

This is the story of Heather and myself, from the very beginning to the end that came way too soon. I will be extremely honest, and at times, very angry. I did my best to remember all the important information. People die in many different ways, and so we grieve in many different ways. This is just one of many stories in this world. For those of you who are reading this because you are feeling the loss of a loved one, I hope this book helps you to heal just a little. I believe it helped me to write it.

I'd also like to thank all the people at the Wellness Community-Foothills, for all their support and understanding that Heather and myself received. They helped us to not **feel** alone in our fight with cancer. They also helped me to not **feel** alone after Heather died.

Chapter 1
How we met, and our relationship.

The very first time we went out was when we where in high school. We where in our junior year, if I remember correctly. It was 1988. We where set up by a mutual friend of ours, Alina. Alina thought we would hit it off because we both played the drums. I was a teenage boy and Heather was something of a tomboy. I was hormone driven and she was not. We got along O.K., but there was no spark, despite her natural beauty. She had natural copper red hair, heavenly blue eyes, a happy smile, and a soothing voice, and mildly freckled pale skin. She was that tomboy **hot** that an eighteen-year-old would fantasize about. She was sixteen and, other than drums, and a love for the same style of music, we didn't hit it off like our friend thought we would. We went out just a few times, and then stopped calling each other.

Over the next few years, I would see her around at the community college we went to and at an A.T.M once. Each time I thought she was looking good and thought of asking her out. But I was steady with another girl, so nothing was ever acted on.

I broke-up with the other girl in '93. Then, around 1996, I was at a pool hall with Alina and a friend of hers that we knew. We where playing pool and Heather walked in with another friend, Francine, to find Frans' boyfriend. She saw me and came over to say "Hi." Again, she was looking good and dumb ass me didn't get her phone number. Well about two weeks later I was gonna go Karaoke singing with Alina and some friends she said she had invited. So I get to her apartment and a few minuets later, in walks Heather!!!!!!!!!! She came strait up to me to say hello, and little did I know my life would change forever. For the rest of the night, we where inspirable. We had so much fun! After that we went back to Alinas' apartment. Now I don't quite remember the whole "bases" code, but I think we went to second base. When I took her home, we sat in front of her house till 5am talking. I only left because she said her dad was going to wake up to go to work and she had to get in the house. We went to a late breakfast with Alina and Heathers' younger brother Dennis. We saw each other every night for a week. She was still tomboy hot, and this time we where really into each other.

Now Heather later told me that she wanted to get my phone number when she saw me at the pool hall, but was too shy to ask. She wanted to call Alina to get it, but didn't. Perhaps Alina saw something between us and arranged the situation, I don't know, but I'm glad it happened.

Then I had to go to a camp that I volunteered for, for a week. I wrote her a letter from camp. That was a big deal for me because I <u>never</u> wrote to anyone form camp. When I came back, we where going out every night again for a week. Then I went to another two camps for two weeks. This time

I called her several times, and wrote. A good friend of mine from one of these camps, was a guy named Eric. He later told me he knew I had found someone special when he saw that I was calling her from camp during fellowship.

Heather had an older sister, Carolyn, and four brothers, Patrick, Brian, and Sean where older than her, and Dennis, the youngest. Her parents are Betty and Larry. The family was, and still is, into a lot of friendly 'ribbing'. While I was gone at camp, they had some fun at her sister's house. Carolyn, Liz,(Heathers' niece), and her friend Fran taped themselves dressing up, putting on some wild make up, and lip sinking to disco tunes for fun.

So when I got back from camp, they thought it would be fun to show me the video. Heather was mortified. I thought it was great!! This woman really knew how to have fun. I told her it was funny and I liked it. Not long after that, we decided that we wanted to just date each other. Everyday we fell further in love with each other. For a little while, we where both unemployed. Instead of being depressed, we just figured we had more time to spend together. I was accepted into the McCarthy family as if I where one of the boys. We finally got jobs, and for about two years, even worked together. This just made us even happier.

In the first couple of months that we went out, a band called Oingo Boingo had a C.D. singing at Tower Records on Sunset Blvd. Now Heather was a Boingo fanatic! She had an obsession with Danny Elfman that was just short of stalking. So we went and got the whole bands autographs on a shirt of the last tour, and the double live C.D. that came out. For our first Christmas in our house, I had those items framed to put in a room that was our office/Boingo shrine. There are various other Boingo items in the room too. She was so excited about seeing the band, and Elfman that she told me later that she peed "just a little bit" in her pants.

Shortly after this I heard that her family and friends called her Beaner. This was because when she was a kid, she got a bean stuck up her nose.

They called her Heather bean, or Beaner for short.

Another funny memory was at the local mall. We went to the See's candy store and got some truffles. The one that she got had a cherry in it, filled with some heavenly goo. As we walked in the mall, we came to an area that had a good echo to it. Just then, the bag slipped out of my hand and hit the floor. When I picked it up to see if our treats where destroyed, she looked at me and asked in a very concerned, and loud voice, "Did you pop my cherry?!" I instantly started laughing and she looked confused, not realizing what she said, or how it sounded. Then she noticed that most people in that area of the mall had turned to hear the rest of what was to be said. Then it all hit her and she tuned beat red, smiled and started laughing too.

Then in ë99, we got an apartment together. By this time we no longer worked together, and I even quit my job at one point. Now we never argued, or had a "heated" discussion. Not even at this time! We just lived our lives for each other, and to see the other smile. I found some more jobs and things where great. We kept our money separate, but still shared everything as if what was mine was hers and what was hers was mine. Our relationship was one of balance.

We completed each other.

We had what the other needed, and added more of what we already had.

This was the year people started to ask us about marriage. I had my own lame reasons not to get married and she would just tell people, "He'll ask me when he's ready." She **never** pushed the issue. As far as we where concerned, we where the happiest couple on the planet! I was her "bubbie" and she was just "beautiful" to me. We where the happiest couple to ever live.

As it turned out, my parents where moving to another city to live for their retirement. They asked if Heather and I would like to move into the house. We said yes because my parents where kind enough to charge us cheaper rent. So in January of 2000, we moved into my old house. To help make her more comfortable, I told her she could decorate the house any way she wanted to. This was also because any idea I would come up with would be so out there, that people would probably never come to see us. Things where just peachy.

In November of 2000, I decided my lame reasons for not getting married where no match for making the woman that I loved happy. I wanted to live out our lives as husband and wife. So I went to the jewelry store to get us engagement rings.

It wasn't a fancy ring. She didn't like fancy jewelry. (lucky me) It was just a simple white gold band. (she didn't like yellow gold) I wanted to surprise her on Christmas. We would always try to get the other as many gifts as possible, so I didn't think she would see a ring and proposal coming. She told me later that she knew I was going to propose. She claimed woman's intuition. Heather and I met eachother just as we where both at the same "station" in our lives. We found our joy and happiness in eachother. Our means of escaping all the bad things was to be with eachother. Our hearts and souls where the same, so we found "home" in eachother. I'll always be greatful for our love, and the strength she helped me see in myself.

Chapter 2
The diagnosis, proposal, and treatments.

In late October of 2000, Heather started to get really bad headaches. She'd get them more often in the next two months. On December 19th, I was at band rehearsal when I got a call on my cell phone from Dennis. He told me Heather was being taken to the hospital. After he told me which one, I told the guys in the band that I had to go. Driving to the hospital, all kinds of things went through my head. It was the most worried I'd ever been.

When I got to the emergency room, Betty and Larry, Dennis, and I think Carolyn, where there. They told me that she called her parent's house and Dennis answered. She sounded confused and must have dropped the phone. Dennis told Betty and Larry, and they rushed over to the house. They saw her through the front window lying on the floor. Dennis got in through the back window and held her, as she was semiconscious. He talked to her as her mom called the ambulance.

When I went in to see her, she said she tried to call me, but wound up calling her parents. She said she felt very strange, as if separate from her body.

Then the room felt as if it where spinning, then things got dim. The next thing she knew, Dennis was holding her, sitting on the floor, and she had trouble talking. She told me later that she looked at Dennis as her hero for getting into the house and holding her.

The doctors tested her blood, found nothing and said she needed to rest and eat better. This was on a Tuesday. The next day, she made an appointment with her doctor for that Friday. Thursday, the 21st was my birthday and we went out to eat. She had not been feeling write since Tuesday. We both thought that she had some sort of deficiency in her body chemistry, yet the blood work at the E.R. showed nothing.

Friday, December 22nd, 2000. I went to work, and she went to the doctor. At around 9am I got a call from her mother on my cell. She said Heather had a grandmal seizure in the doctor's exam room and was being taken to the hospital. I told the people at my work what had happened, I didn't ask to leave, I just left. Not to cool since I worked with people that have developmental disabilities. We where out in the community, and I just took off. They where still under supervision from other staff, but I left them shot handed.

When I got to the hospital, I went to the emergency room to see her. She looked tired and told me her doctor said she probably had epilepsy. The doctors this time did a "cat scan" and didn't like what they saw, so they did an M.R.I. Of coures all this took hours to get done, She was admitted to the E.R. at around 10am and the M.R.I was done at around 9pm. At around 10pm or later, we where in an E.R. bed jokingly saying, *"It's not a toomar,"* like Arnold Schwarzenegger.

We'll when the doctor came in to tell us what the results where, another one came in and wanted to talk to the first one outside the Curtin. We could hear her telling the other doctor; "Did you see the M.R.I results?" A few words later they both came in and told us she had a brain tumor. She was 28 years old.

No words can describe how I felt. I was holding her hand, gave it kiss and waited for her reaction. All she had was disbelief and a "So what's next" attitude. From what I remember, Betty and Carolyn where there to, and just as devastated as I was. I didn't cry. This was because I wanted to be strong for her. I thought if I didn't look too distraught, she might not take it as bad, and not cry. She was admitted to the hospital that night, and was scheduled to have a biopsy just a day or two after Christmas.

I still felt I wanted to marry her. I had the engagement rings, and still felt the same way. I truly wanted to be her husband. It's hard to put into words, but I wasn't going to let a thing like cancer spoil our lives.

Well they kept her pretty doped up to keep the seizures under control. On Christmas I went to the hospital to give her some of her gifts, and to propose. She opened the few gifts I brought and we told each other "I love you." Then I said "oh, I forgot I have this other little present for you." I pulled out the small box with the ring in it. She opened it and looked at me. I looked at her and said," Heather, I love you so much. Will you marry me?" She said "yes" and made me the happiest guy on the planet. We hugged and kissed, and where a bit giddy. Then a nurse walked in and asked, "Did I just hear you propose to her?" We said yes and then he asked if he was the first to know. I told him he was, but not for long, I was going to go and call our parents soon. We sat for a little longer looking at our rings and each other. I said some words to make her strong and said I'd go call our parents and be right back.

Our moms cried when I called them, and I asked them to call the rest of our families so I could get back to Heather.

Later that morning I went to the McCarthy home for Christmas breakfast.

The morning of the 29th, she had her biopsy. The surgeons needed to drill a very small hole in her skull to insert some kind of probe to take a small sample of the tumor. This was done to determine what kind of cancer was causing the tumor, so they could figure out what kind of treatment to give her.

Now we where never told what "grade" the tumor was, but later we learned it was a 4. This is on a scale with 5 being the worst. It had been growing for five years according to the doctors.

The type she had was an *Oligodenrogliomas*, or an 'oligo', for short. It was deep in the brain, in the cerebrum, next to the Corpus callosum, on the right side of her brain. This tumor dose not "branch out into the brain. It dose keep expanding and puts pressure on the brain, causing your life to be greatly inconvenienced. In looking at the M.R.I.'s, I felt so many things, anger, frustration, sadness, and a general feeling of being overwhelmed. I put all this aside to help Heather the best I could, any way I could. The one up side, we where told, is that this tumor responds well to chemo, and if she *had* to have a tumor, this was the one to get. *Oh, fucking joy!* We decided to wait a year while we plan the wedding and

Heather goes through her treatment. When she got back from the hospital, she didn't remember me proposing. She was standing next to the bed and looking at the ring. She told me "I know we're engaged, but I don't remember you asking." So I got down on one knee and asked again. She said yes again, and we forgot about the cancer for a few minutes. I used to joke about how that was my chance to get out of the whole wedding, and I blew it!

One of the ways to help her was to keep track of her various medications she was on, and to look out for the side affects. There where quite a few of each, and I always kept an updated list of the medications, in various easy to access places. This was just in case anything happened; the paramedics had all the pertinent information. This came in handy numerous times during her illness.

One of the things we had to deal with was the fact that the tumor would cause a "focal" seizure. This was a seizure that would cause intense pain, and at times spasms, in her left foot. They where on the left side because the tumor was on the right side of the brain.

Do to all the various medications she was on, the side affects where just as numerous.

Anything from, disorientation, nausea, joint pain, dizziness, rashes, discordination, and as with all of them, fatigue!!! At any given time she was on at least six different medications. All to help her, despite the side affects. All of it **sucked**, but it gave me a focus, a purpose, to keep me occupied and to look out for her the best I could. All I could do was to make things as easy as possible, tolerable, for her. This goal was not always achieved due to the nature of the illness, but it helped the both of use get through things.

Also, because of the stress of the situation, we would "snap" at each other, from time to time. We would both apologize, knowing it was the cancer at the root of the anger.

The first doctor we talked to told us the usual procedure was to first surgically remove as much of the tumor as possible. Well, this being her brain and all, we said we where going to get another opinion. We did. When it comes to things like this and just your bodies in general, don't be scared to get another opinion. As we came to see things, the doctors are your employees'. You can trust them, but make sure you feel they are making the right decision for **you.** In our case, the other doctor had a better idea as to how we could start treatment.

This was good because the original doctor told us he had never seen a brain tumor before! Apparently they are a rare form of cancer, and most doctors haven't seen them, even though they are becoming more common. This second doctor was not approved by her H.M.O to give treatment, so we had the original doctor give the treatment prescribed by the second. Most of the time, we had to fight tooth and nail to get cretin things to happen, to get treatments, meds, second opinions, etc., but if you look at it as an opportunity to harass them for not looking out for your best interest, it's kind of fun. Also, it helps you to vent a bit. Getting what you need is a big plus too. Just remember that no amount of complaining can make the situation go away, and can possibly make things worse. I'd also like to thank my parents. They "know people" in the medical industry that where of great help in finding out if a doctor had a good reputation or not. They also got us set up with a patient advocate with the H.M.O that Heather was with. I'd suggest to anyone that has trouble with his or her heath care provider, to look for one. Independently, or with your H.M.O.

The first chemo was called P.V.C for short. It was to be injected, numerous times over an eight-month period, starting in February of 2001.

During this time there where various trips to the hospital for various reasons. None of which was a pleasant experience. The majority of them happening at very early hours of the morning. Effects of the chemo, too much of a build up of certain medications, and just effects of the tumor where most of the causes. I still can't remember all the situations, or all the facts. Can't say I want to either. One constant was the pain she would get in her knees due to the mass amount of steroids she was on. She had to take them to keep the swelling around the tumor to a minimum. She would wake up at around 4 or 5am with the intense pain and nothing would make it go away. Not even the painkillers she got. After a few hours, the pain would stop.

During this time as well, she had to stop working. Her doctors considered her disabled and the focal seizure activity was not under control. It was extremely hard for her to get on SSI, disability. She finally did and it helped her pay her bills and the co-pays when she went to the hospital, which was a lot! It was a lot of unnecessary stress and just another hassle to deal with on top of the tumor.

In the fist few months, I'd say till about April, she was in a denial almost. She took her meds and went to the doctors, but it never really sank in that she had cancer.

One day we where on the couch, in the living room, discussing what to do about our money situation. I told her I'd figure something out and that I just wanted her to concentrate on getting better. I told her "you have cancer" and that she needed to be concerned with her treatment above all else. Just then she started crying uncontrollably. After a few minutes, she told me she hadn't truly realized it, till I said it. We just held each other for a while.

Lots of things happened that made our situation a bit easier, if you could say that. Just one of them was having my parents as "landlords." They immediately told us to not worry about the rent till Heather was able to work again. If we where still in the apartment, I'm sure we would have had to move out.

Heathers' parents and the rest of the family helped out a great deal too. I couldn't make most of her appointments, so they would go with her. When I had rehearsals with my band, they would come to keep her company, or she could go to them.

I never realized how devastating cancer could be till I had to deal with it on a personal level. With someone I truly loved. One of the other deeply sad moments was when Heather had to give up her driver's license, due to her seizures not being under control. Whenever she cried, I'd cry with her.

She was only 28 when she was diagnosed. She only had her license for a few months, and now she was unemployed, had to take all kinds of medications that made her feel like shit, and lost so much of her independents. Not just the license, but the ability to feel safe when left alone. At any time her body could turn on her and she couldn't do jack shit about it! Neither could I.

We where told that one of the side affects of the chemo was the loss of hair. She had a lot of hair, and she lost a lot of it when I combed it out after her showers. You would have never known. Her hair was so thick; you could not tell that I was pulling large amounts of it out when I combed it.

In October, the chemo was over and we waited to hear what the next step would be. She still had to take all the medications. In November, we where told that the tumor had not grown, but did not shrink either. They where to come up with another chemo treatment that she was to go on. Well, December came around, and no plan yet. On my birthday, almost a year to the day of her first seizure, she had another grandmal seizure. So, off to the E.R. we go, yet again, and with allot more concern. She had not had another grandmal since the original one a year earlier. This obviously did not look like a good thing.

Another M.R.I was done, and it showed that the tumor had grown! We thought *what the fuck! You guys said it stopped growing!* She was admitted to the hospital again, for a short time. Then a surgery was scheduled for January 2nd of 2002.

This time they where going to cut a piece of her skull out and go into the brain, and take as much of the tumor out as possible. A pretty tricky maneuver when in the brain. This news **fucking sucked** to say the least. At least she was home for Christmas this time. Little did I know that this was our last Christmas together.

At the end of the surgery, the surgeon came out to tell us he felt the tumor had changed to something worse. He said he wanted to wait for the pathology report to be sure.

About a week later, we went to hear what the doctor had to say and to get the staples out of Heathers head. Her mom, sister and sister-in-law, Melissa came with us. Well, it wasn't good. The pathology report confirmed what he had suspected. The tumor had changed to a Glioblastoma. It was a multiform because it still had some of the original tumor cells in it. This was **bad**. He said she could have radiation, and some more chemotherapy, and that would give her 18 months.

We went to the waiting room afterward and digested a little more of what we where told. I told Heather I still wanted to marry her and we could move the wedding date up. Then we all had a good cry. She said she wanted to go through the treatments and we moved the wedding date up. It was originally set for July 27, 2002. We moved it to May 24.

In February of 2002, she started her radiation. It took the rest of her hair in about a week. She had radiation for about a month and a half. At the end of it all, the tumors had just multiplied. She now had five instead of one. Three in the frontal lobe, the original, and one right next to the original.

Chapter 3
The wedding

During all the treatments, one of the things that kept her occupied and looking forward, was the wedding and planning it. I just wanted to get married and didn't really care about the specifics. I let her plan what ever she wanted and would answer her questions and help in any way she would ask me.

We went to a place in New Port beach that had boats for weddings. We got the Idea from her brother Brian and his wife Melissa. They had their wedding with the same company just about two years before. It was kind of a package deal. This worked out for us because it was easy to find the photographer and the D.J. from the company's referrals. Also, they did the catering. We found our photo guy and the D.J. Later our parents picked the food; this was due to her not being up for it at the time because of her treatments. Our parents helped a lot with the planning and other things when we needed them to. They paid for the whole thing too. *That was a major help. Thanks to both our parents for all their help.* We where able to go to the wedding cake place and get her ideal cake.

Now Heathers oldest brother Pat was not a part of the other two weddings in her family, Carolyn or Brian's.

So we decided to ask him and his "husband" Dave to get ordained over the Internet, so they could marry us! They where both happy that we asked and said they would do it. To get ordained on the Internet was easy. I even did it!

When we went to get our license, she was feeling weak that day. Her sister got her a wheel chair a few months before, and unfortunately we put it to good use. So I wheeled her in to the building and we got the license. To get the wedding rings, we went to a few places. Mine was easy to pick, hers wasn't hard, but took a few places to go to. She got a bit tired again, and we used the wheel chair, *again*. I felt really bad having to wheel my fiancé' around. Not that it was her fault, but because of the situation and I felt bad that she couldn't walk like she used to. I felt that she didn't get the ring that she really wanted, due to the money situation. She insisted that she was happy with what she got. I told her we had the money to get her a better ring, but she said she liked the one we got just fine.

We made the list of whom we wanted to see at the wedding and then gave it to our parents to add who they wanted to have. When it was all done, and all the replies came back, we had about one hundred guests.

That worked out fine for the boat, and us as well too.

Heather went with her sister, her niece Liz, Francine, and I'm not sure whom else, to get her dress and the brides' maid dresses. Heather saw the one she wanted right away! The other girls got the dresses that they all liked. Apparently a big deal for bride's maids. All where happy. As far as myself, and my guys, it's pretty easy to get a tux. We got a deal for seven tuxedos. We couldn't all try the tuxedos on before we picked them up, so not every ones fit well, but we all looked sharp.

Carolyn was Heathers brides' maid, and Liz and Fran finished the rest of her court. I had my cousin Mark as my best man, and my uncle Dan and a good friend Steve finished my court.

The night before the wedding, a lot of us stayed at a hotel in New Port beach. We had dinner and other guests arrived to stay the night before as well. We all talked and had a good time. Heather and I where never nervous. People would ask us all the time and we always said no. It just seemed so natural of a thing that there was no anxiety at all about anything. We just wanted to have all the arrangements taken care of on time. That night I wrote my vows to Heather before going to bed.

The Day of The Wedding
May 24, 2002

Everything was good! The wedding was in the evening, so we had a pretty relaxing day. More guests came to stay at the hotel, and Heather and I still had some moments alone before she had to get ready. When the time came to get ready, her court came in and did their thing with her to help her to get ready. Heather wrote her vows to me while getting ready.   Now, at this point, Heather had all her radiation. She had lost all her hair. So she had gone out and found a wig. I wasn't sure how a wig would look and I told her I was good with her just having a head wrap of some nice material. She wanted to go with the wig. When I got to see her, she still looked beautiful. The girls did a great job in making her look good for her wedding. The whole wedding party looked good.

The singer and main writer of the band I was in, Zach, is a director, and did our wedding video, at our request. He got some really good footage and did a great job editing it. I stood around the boat and greeted a lot of the guests that came on, along with our parents. Heather just rested in the room she had on the boat and let the people come to her.

The ceremony was great! This is in a great part to Pat and especially Dave. It started at 6pm as the sun was going down for the evening.

We picked out our own music. Heather used a song from Queen, "It's a beautiful day" to walk down the aisle to. We had a couple of readings, and then we exchanged our vows.

Mine where, "Heather, when I met you, I finally realized what true love was. I realized I wanted to share the rest of our lives together. The compassion and bravery you've shown me has humbled me and made me a better person. I'm lucky to become your husband today. I love you." Now this didn't come out as smooth as I had hoped it would, mainly because I was crying after the first sentence. I was told later that had made a lot of other people cry too. Every one at the wedding knew Heathers situation.

There was some laughter as I handed the microphone to Heather because she didn't realize that it was her turn to speak. Her vows where simple. She wrote them that day.

"Mike, my best friend and true love. I stand here in front of you today and give you myself entirely."

With that, Pat pronounced us husband and wife, and we walked down the isle to another Queen tune called, "I was born to love you." The wedding photos where taken as the reception was being set up. I helped her down the steps to the lower level for the cake cutting.

All the flashes that went off seemed like it was the stalk-eratzzi.

We went back up for the reception, and my cousins toast. I cried for that too! Man what a blubber head I was.

We did the dances with our parents, and our first dance as husband and wife. Then the party began. Heather danced just a little bit and got to tired to continue. So she sat and watched every one have a great time. Looking back now I feel bad that she couldn't participate more, but she did have a good time. She said she liked watching everyone having fun.

I watched the video alot after she died, and still watch it on our anniversary now, and it still makes me cry. But that's o.k, she was my wife and I'll always miss her.

For our honeymoon, we went to Hawaii. Specifically the island of Molokai. All we really did was rest and lounge and eat and enjoy each other's company. We had lots of memories to take home of funny things that had happened on the trip, and Heather was looking forward to opening all the wedding gifts we got.

I remember when we got to the big island and had to take an island hopper. It was only her third plane ride. She asked why we didn't have seat numbers on the tickets.

I told her they had to pick our seats to balance the plane.

She thought I was kidding and I had a good laugh when she realized I was not kidding.

She was a bit jumpy around birds too, and the wild turkeys on the beach made things fun.

When we returned, it was back to trying another chemotherapy treatment.

Chapter 4
Heather's Death

We got back from our honeymoon in June. She tried another type of chemo treatment. This was to give her a chance at extending her time into 2003. June and July went on with her physical condition getting worse. Her walking had been bad since she started the radiation, now it was getting worse. She would drop things and couldn't hold on to stuff like she used too. She would forget a lot of things and had to be watched by some one in the family while I was at work. As bad as this seemed, I still thought we actually had till some time next year. One night in August, we watched T.V. till late at night. When I got up to go to bed, she seemed really tiered. I told her to come to bed soon. She mumbled something, not unusual at this point, and I went to bed. The next morning she was still on the couch. When her mom came to be with her for the day, I told her the situation, and went to work. A couple of hours later I got a call from Betty telling me that she tried to get Heather up and put her in bed. She had trouble and realized she had to call the ambulance.

I met them at the hospital. Heather was unconscious in the E.R. room.

I sat beside her and held her hand. She had gained about 20 pounds from the medications she was on, and when a nurse had to insert a catheter, she asked about her stretch marks. I explained the situation and she just said, "poor girl." I don't know why this stands out in my memory, but it dose.

When the M.R.I came back, it showed that the tumors had gotten larger and where starting to exert too much pressure on her brain. They admitted her, and we took the films to the doctor we had the most confidence in. He said she could try one last chemo option, but she had only three more months. Staring at the M.R.I films, I started crying. Carolyn was with me and we cried together.

I went back to the hospital to tell Heather. This was almost a week after she was admitted. She was awake and had a lot of medication. I told her she had about three months to live and it was suggested to have hospice care at the house. She past on the chemo that was suggested, and I asked her what she wanted me to do with her after she died. This shred' my soul to ask. I had to ask twice to make sure she knew what I was saying. She said she wanted to be cremated, and have her ashes spread in the ocean. I put my head in her lap and cried and she just held me. She told me not to let her family push me into anything I didn't want.

She also said she didn't want a religious ceremony. A few days later she was at home.

Her godmother, Judy, had hired a lady to stay with Heather and I during the week. This was so I could go to work and have some help with Heather if things got too hard. The weekends it was just her family and us. That week, Pat and

Dave took me to a friend of theirs who ran a mortuary. They said they'd pay for the expenses, and the arrangements where made.

The first day she was home, we took a shower together. I helped her wash herself and to stand, and then sit, in the shower. I took her back to the bed after that. It was the last time she stood up and walked at all. The next day her legs didn't have the strength to hold her up. This was because the tumors where interfering with her motor skills. She was very shaky, and uncoordinated since she got back from the hospital. More so than before.

She was also acting very angry and uncoperatetive. This was primarily due to the three tumors in the frontal lobe of her brain. That is the area that controls behavior. We where given **a lot** of medications to give her for her comfort, help her control herself, and feel less pain. For a while she was able to take them with water, in pill form.

After a few weeks, I had to crush them and put them in a "shake" type of drink.

The first weekend she was back, she had a temperature of 102.9. I called her family because I knew they would want to be there if this was the end. All we could do was treat her with ice and wipe her down with cool water, and give her aspirin. Her pupils where not even. One was small and the other was wide open. She was semiconscious and could barley answer questions. She had singed a D.N.R (do not recessitate) order. But that was the whole point of being on hospice care, to wait to die. I felt the most helpless I ever felt till this point. This started late on a Friday night and went on till Monday night. Her temperature went up and down. She was still able to eat when her tempt went down at times, but needed help eating. Any time I was home I did every thing I could for her. I felt bad feeding her, this wasn't what we planned. We where suppose to grow old together. Now I'm watching my wife waiting to die. **This fucking sucked!!** By Tuesday her temperature went back to normal.

I remember leaving for work and looking at her in the hospice bed in the living room. Some times she would be in the recliner chair, looking out the window. She would touch the window when our dog, Jake, came up to it to see her.

Velcro, her cat would be by her side a lot. When I'd get home, she would be asleep. She'd wake up for dinner and stay up for awhile. I slept in the living room, on the couch, next to her so I could be near her, and to help her in the night, if she needed it. She didn't talk much. I wanted to know what she was going through so I could be that outlet for her.

I would also lay next to her in her bed, so we could be close. I'd wash her feet, that always made her feel better before, so I figured it would now too.

We took her out to dinner once. We had to use the damm wheel chair. Again, not her fault, but upset me any way. I'd take her to sit out side to the front of the house. I also would wheel her up and down the street in front of the house. The lady who helped us would do this to.

This went on from late August to October. Heathers' 30th birthday was Oct. 17, 2002. Numerous friends and acquaintances came to celebrate. They all brought small gifts and cards and smiles. Every one knew that was her last birthday. I would read her cards to her, and had a very difficult time holding back the tears. I did manage to do so for her benefit. I didn't want her to feel any worse than she probably did already. Yet I could tell we felt each other's sadness. I did my best to mingle and talk with people, but stayed by her side most of the night.

It was around this time I took my vacation time from work.

For the past two weeks her shaking continued to get worse. Her pupils wear not even either. She was in a lot of pain, with headaches and lots of joint pain from the steroids. She would wake up often during the night and I would get her the pain medication she needed. This was not an unusual thing since she started with the steroids. She had also lost the ability to speak. We would ask her questions and she'd answer by nodding her head, shaking it, or blinking her eyes. She could still squeeze my hand a bit too.

October 26th. She didn't wake up to take her meds, in an Ensure "shake", by now she had great difficulty swallowing her pills for the past month. Her jaw was closed tight, she didn't respond to any stimulation. She would shake on her left side and her pupils where noticeably different sizes. For the past two days she couldn't squeeze my hand. From time to time she would let out a moan, and had difficulty breathing. On the 27th around 2:15 am, she had alot of seizure activity for several hours. This continued for the next day.

Late in the evening on Sunday the 27th, her temperature went up again. I called her family like before.

We all just sat and tried to comfort her the best we could with ice and cool cloths. After a few hours we stopped the treatment and let things take their course. We all sat around her and I gave her some Oxygen that the hospice provided because she was having trouble breathing. At around 2am on that Monday morning, she opened her eyes. At this time her parents Betty and Larry, Carolyn and her husband, Liz, Judy, and my mom where by her bedside. I whispered all the love I could to her and we looked at each other. I held her hand and told her not to be scared. She would look around the bed and see every one, even Velcro the cat was laying beside her. I kissed her cheek and stroked her head and things continued on like this for a few minutes. I whispered in her ear things that I hoped would ease her mind and make things less scary. At one point she looked at me and tried to say something. I said, "*I love you to.*" After about a minute I told her it was O.K. and "*We're ready when you are.*" I said this one more time and she slowly stopped breathing. Just as she took her last couple breaths, I told her "*I love you, I'll see you later, it's O.K.*" With that she stopped breathing, at 2:15 am, it was a Monday morning. We all cried for the next few minutes, and then called the rest of the family that had gone home just a few hours earlier. We also had to call the hospice nurse to come and pronounce the death, and the mortuary to come and get her body. She was cremated that Wednesday, and the memorial was that Friday. For the next six months, I felt an intens emotional pain, or numbness, or pure anger, nothing els.

So many people came to the memorial, that some where literally outside in the lobby and in front of the mortuary. We had some flowers and her ashes up front with some photo albums for people to look at.

I started the memorial by thanking every one for coming, and by reading a poem I wrote the day after she died. It
wasn't up beat, or inspirational. It was just my feelings at that
moment. The following is what I wrote.

There's so much she wanted to do

So much she hasn't done

But she did know true love

And that's a lot for a woman her age

She showed me bravery that humbles me

And had compassion that stuns me still

We spent over six years together

And I got to marry my best friend

In her last moments, she was surrounded by

What meant the most to her, her family.

As I whispered all the love in the universe to her

I knew she was going to a place where she would
be the happiest she's ever been

We'll all feel her love, and she'll feel ours

As long as we remember her, she'll live on

As long as we can tell her stories
and laugh and smile and say her name

She'll live with us

When I was done, I told the "cherry" story and got a good laugh from every one. I then invited anyone to come up and share a story about Heather.

I do not remember the order, but I think my parents came up and my dad read this:

When Mike and Heather were first dating, six years ago, we would notice how compatible they were. They were mostly quiet about their relationship, however, we figured that she was the one for him, after noticing all those loving looks they gave each other and how much they cared for each other.

For a short period of time, they even worked together at the local Shell Station.

Heather as the cashier and Michael in the service area. They were in 7th heaven working together. I would pull up to the gas pump and Heather would look over to Mike and lovingly say "Mikey, someone at the pump." Of course, it helped having a good boss that created a good working enviornment......... Thanks, Bob, for those days!

In December of 2000, Mike had made his mind up to marry Heather and was planning to propose to her on Christmas of that year. Approx. a week before Christmas, Heather was in the hospital being diagnosed with a brain tumor. Mike proposed to Heather later that day. These two beautiful people knew the meaning of "**for better or for worse, in sickness and**

in health....untill death do us part" even before they were officially married.

Mike and Heather were like soul mates. They were literally "two peas in a pod". They brought out the best in each other. We admired Heather for her strength, her beauty, her courage, her smartness, and so many other things. She deeply loved Michael and he deeply loved her. Their love for each other was very apparent even through all their ordeals. What role models they were! We could not help but admire both of them.

Heather became our daughter-in-law on May 24th of this year, however we considered her as **our daughter** even before that time. Her life was very short on this earth, but she brought so much joy and love during this period, that we could not help but admire her.

We gratefully acknowledge the McCarthy family for their unfailing efforts especially during those last few days. A special thanks to Judy. (Heather's second mom) and to Elsie (her caretaker).

There is a big void in Michael's life that will probably never be filled, however, he is also full of her love that will never be forgotten. Michael is the best son anyone could ever have, but as he said in his vows to her at their wedding..."you made me a better man..." Heather did just that and we loved her dearly. We will truly miss her.

I'd like to thank my parents for those words and the sentiment behind them. To have my parents say that they admired us was..., well, wow! The next to come up was her brother Brian, and his wife Melissa. She read this:

Heather Bean was the 5th of 6 children in the McCarthy family. She grew up in Eagle Rock and attended St. Dominic's Catholic school from 1st through 8th grades. In 3rd grade, she stuck a bean up her nose, and earned the nickname Heather Bean from that day onward.

During her high school years, Heather and her best girlfriend Nicky shared many happy times and were always there to support each other. In fact, when Heather needed to attend night school to graduate, Nicky went to class with her even though she didn't need to go herself. And as true friends often do, Heather was there for Nicky when Nicky needed a place to call home. These two friends went on to graduate from high school at Eagle Rock High School in 1990 together.

Like most of us, Heather held several jobs. She first started working at 31 Flavors in the Eagle Rock mall and the Save-On shopping center, and then at B. Dalton Bookstore in the Pasadena Plaza. From there she took a job as a kindergarten assistant in Ms. Chris Borra's class at Precious Blood Catholic Elementary School, and later was hired as a Service Representative for Bank of America.

Heather was interested in, supported, and volunteered for community activities and issues related to the prevention and treatment of HIV and AIDS. This cause was very near and dear to her heart. She looked forward to contributing to the work of APLA each year by participating in the annual AIDS walk fundraiser, and other local community events. She believed in giving her time to help others even if she didn't know them personally. When she needed support from her community, she received it through the Wellness Community Foundation in Pasadena. She was devoted to her cancer support group that she attended regularly.

Heather loved the ocean, camping, fishing, and music (her favorite drummer was Mike). She always looked forward to our annual Mammoth family camping trip so that she could get in some good trout fishing with her brother Brian. Most of all, she loved our family game nights. Some of her favorite games were Murder, Hide and Seek, Cranium, Dominos, and Monopoly. In fact, she hosted one of the best Murder nights we ever had at mom and dads. Heather liked to have fun! Even as an adult, she never forgot the importance of play and fun.

Heather was a very casual person. She didn't like to wear dresses, or get dressed up for that matter. She preferred her jeans and t-shirt, wearing no make-up and a ponytail; yet she radiated a natural beauty with her bright copper red hair and sparkling blue eyes.

Heather was the kind of person that could capture a room with her story telling. She was quick witted, animated, and quite humorous. Even if she were telling you a story for the fifth time, you would still laugh as if it was the first. Her alter ego must have been part actress, because on occasion, she would dress up in outlandish costumes and make-up and lip sink and dance to her favorite disco tunes during dress up nights at Carolyn's.

Heather was an easy person to talk to and a good listener. She was the kind of person that you could immediately feel relaxed around. That's probably one of the reasons why it was so easy for people to like her so quickly. And seeing you all hear today is proof of that to us.

Heather's life revolved around the two most important things to her in all the world-her family and her soul mate Mike. Some people spend their whole lives striving to attain material wealth and riches, but Heather, at age 30, was wealthy beyond measure because she possessed the support, devotion, and love of this very special group of people- Mom, Dad, Patrick, Brian, Carolyn, Sean, Dennis, Liz, Gary, Dave, Kelly, Cecilia and Irv, Judy (her second mom) and myself, and the greatest love in her lifetime, her husband Mike.

On behalf of our family, we want to extend our deepest, heartfelt appreciation to each person here, both family and friends, that have enjoyed good times with her, shared happy memories, supported, and loved Heather, our daughter, wife, sister, friend.

Love, Melissa

After that, I think her friend John came up to talk. I believe her friend Francine, and her brother Sean came up to. When it was over, we had some music that she liked play as every one just hung out for a bit and talked, and looked at the photo albums. My uncle Danny has a fishing boat, so I figured I would ask him what I needed to rent a boat, so I could take her ashes to the ocean. He said he was willing to take me, but he could only fit six people on the boat.

In December, I think, we had the opportunity, to go and take her ashes out to the ocean. We went up the coast, about 1000 yards off shore of a beach my uncle knew about, and that would be a nice place to visit. The trip up was short and it was a nice day. Carolyn, Dennis, Liz, Danny and his girl friend Gloria, and myself where there. It was a sunny southern California day and Heather would have enjoyed the whole thing. We stopped, we where quiet, I poured her ashes into the ocean and said "see you later." Carolyn said "bye Heather!" We cried for a little, and Gloria put some flowers in the water. It was all finally done for me. No more worrying anyway.

Chapter 5
Dealing

So, how did we deal with all this? Well, we where pointed in the direction of a place called the Wellness Community. We went to an orientation meeting and they told us of all the different programs, and work shops they had to offer. The first thing we got into was a support group. There was one for the people who where diagnosed, and one for the people that cared for them. Many of these groups where at the same time so both could conviently attend at the same time. A licensed therapist moderates the groups. What is said in the group stays in the group. It was a safe place to vent all my emotions and not feel bad about them. You can complain, cry, and be angry, and laugh. As a result, I felt relieved for that short time and could be more supportive and comforting, since I felt better. I could also share advice with the other people in the group on any thing that they may need help with, and them with me. If I wasn't in a comfortable place in my heart, I couldn't be there for Heather.

Now this would help for a day or two, but then I was left with the rest of the week!

Well, blasting the stereo as LOUD as I could, when I could, really helped a lot! Also playing my drums as often as I could was a big help. Having a band to jam in and some gigs to look forward to was great as well! I would write a lot of poems and songs to. I also realized that there would never be enough ammo in the world to shoot through, but I sure went through a few thousand rounds. (no exaggeration) I read a lot of books and magazines that I'm interested in as well.

Heather got many of the same benefits from her group as well. She also went to some workshops too. She enjoyed them and got a lot out of them. She became very close to some of the people in her group. We both looked forward to going to our groups and getting things off our chest.

As far as my group went, I was the youngest one in it. I was in my early thirties and the next oldest person was in there 50's, the rest of the people where 60 and over. I often herd from the others in the group, that they felt bad for me because they at least got to spend quite a few years with there loved one. When I went to the grievers group after Heather died, I'd hear the same sentiment. Unfortunately, some of the people from my support group ended up in my grievers group too.

We did all the same stuff as the caregiver group did, but as part of a grieving process. I also did all the same stuff I did to deal with my grief as I did when Heather was alive. I also started to paint my old drum heads. I use spray paint and will do some abstract stuff. Once in a while I'll use some brushes, but I like the spray paint better.

One of the things I learned in the group was to not make any major life dissitions for at least a year.

Heather had a life insurance policy, and some stock options through her job. It all added up to quite a few thousand dollars. I pretty much spent all of it. I told myself she would want me to spend it on things that I wanted. Gifts she would have got me if she could've. Should I have saved some of it? Probably! But no money ment no major life dissisions. Spending was a band-aide I needed. I remember seeing things that I knew Heather would've liked, and talking myself out of buying it ëcause she was no longer alive.

When she was alive, I did the best I could to make her physically, and emotionally, comfortable. I'd look on the Internet for any helpful info or hopeful stories. I remember looking at one person's story that was similar to Heathers, they died in the end. Heather walked in and saw me crying.

I told her why and we just held each other and cried together. Some times that was all we needed to do, or could do.

After she died, it was a very dark time for me. Grief can take a big physical toll on you. I never felt more exhausted! I'd cry myself to sleep, and wake up crying, for about a month. I'd cry at any given moment. I've always been one to let feelings come when they do, but these where a lot, all the time. If you fight them, or suppress them, you're only going to feel worse. I was operating on "auto pilot" for a few months. I cann't remember much of that time period. I didn't like to go home either. I would hang out anywhere, just to not be in an empty house with all the memories.

I didn't go to the grievers group right away. It wasn't till about February of 2003. I went because I wasn't dealing with my grief in a way that made me feel good. When I started the group, it felt like a way to move forward.

I felt like I could have done more than I did and especially the last few months. In group, I was told that most people go through those feelings. The adage about hind sight thing fits in hear too. The fact is that I did what I was emotionally ready to do, and my subconscious stopped me at a point where I had to stop.

Another thing we would discuss, was the people who seemed to expect you to "get over it" quicker then you where. It was explained that this attitude was usually due to the fact that your grief reminded them of something they did not want to deal with.

There is knowing that you're not alone, and *feeling* like you're not alone. That is what the Wellness Community did for me. I'll always be grateful for that, and to the people in my group for all the support they gave me. The Wellness Community dose all this for **free**! It was definitely a shining light in a dark period of our lives. I stopped going in March of 2004 because it started to feel as if I was dwelling on the past.

Another help was the support of my family and the McCarthy family, and the guys in my band, and some good friends. I thank all of you.

Another thing that I felt I had to do was to get some of her things together for her brothers and sister, and friends. Each got some items that I felt Heather would've wanted them to have. I hung on to some stuff too. Probably more than I should've, but I'm slowly getting rid of more and just keeping the things that ment the most to me.

I realized that I'd never get "over" Heathers' death. I've talked to a couple of ladies who where widowed at a young age and re-married.

They say they still think of their husbands from time to time, and still miss them. I don't want to forget her, and over the last few years, it stings a lot less to think of her. It dose still hurt, but not like it used to. Our moderator in the grievers group told me that studies showed that the younger one is when losing a spouse, the easier it is to recover from the depression. It took a year and five months till I felt ready to date again. I still say "good night" to her in my own way every night. There are still times I'll cry when I think of her, but I don't cry as much any more. Now I remember the happier times more often, and can smile more. I'll think of her face, her smile, her laugh, her voice, her touch. More of the good times are coming back into my thoughts, and making me smile.

I think of the "cancer" days **a lot** less now. There will still be times in the future when I think of her and cry, but I know now that they will be only at sirten memories and times of the year. For the last three years, I have had a birthday party for Heather. Just as my way to honor her and get everyone together, as she liked it. The McCarthy's get together a lot, but I can't always make it.

There are still times that I think, "Heather would love this!" I just remind myself, she knows and is hear with me.

I had mentioned that I wrote songs and poems, and I'll share a few with you now. The first was written in the first week Heather and I started dating, in July of 1996.

Tomorrow used to be
Just another day for me
Things to, places to go
And people to see
Now you're in my life
Filling my heart with love
Tomorrow is looked forward to
'cause it's another day with you
Looking ahead from time to time
was something I had to do
but now with you
it's what I want to do
Tomorrow and today
can never be too gray
You'll chase the blues away
'cause you're my get away
Thank you for yesterday
Thank you for today
Thank you for tomorrow
and every single day

There's more of my love for her, but I'll just share this one with you. The next two where written after she died.

You brought happiness in a smile

Made life worthwhile

Crying seems to be my past time

As I lay my head down at night

And awake in the morning

Seeing your picture is pleasure and pain

Hearing your voice touches my heart

I hope my words gave you comfort, in the end

We had a good time, after all is said and done

Growin' old with you was my dream

I'm so humbled by you, touched by your soul

Your death took a part of me

And I wanna be whole again, I'll never be

I miss you so, I hope you can see now

You came and went and we had so much fun

In such a short time, I'm so glad you said "yes"

Being rerouted was not the plan, I know

Guess I'll see you again some day, somewhere

I'd just like to say, that if you choose to write in a journal, or songs, or poetry, it dose not matter how good it is, as long as it comes from the heart, you'll feel better. Write for your own well-being and sanity. One more to go.

As you laid on your last bed
We looked into each other's eyes
I held your hand and caressed your skin
And I said, "It's ok to go"
"It's ok, we're ready when you are."

I hope you weren't scared
I know we all cried, 'cause you couldn't stay
All our love was understood
As I kissed you good-bye
And I said, "It's ok to go"
"It's ok, we're ready when you are."
I know you weren't scared
When we cry, it's 'cause we can't wait
To see you again
I know you see us all every day
I know you share the good and bad
And the old and new, with us all
I miss you so
In our hearts and minds

Every day you'll be part of us all

The smile we have

Are your smiles too

And when I "it's ok," I ment it

Whether I like it or not

I know, you know

"It's ok" to go

I'm a better man having known Heather and I'll always be greatfull for the time we had.

Chapter 6
Continuing

So how do I soldier on? I heard a line in a T.V. show in which one man asked another, "How do I go on without her?" The answer was, "Be the man she loved." So I try every day to be that man. In my heart I know she sees me and is happy that I have begun to live my life again and start anew. One thing I've noticed is that everything in my life seems temporary to me now. I'm not sure how to deal with that.

I still keep in contact with my family-in-law. I enjoy seeing my brothers, and my sister, and my other parents. Melissa and Brian have had two baby girls, Meadow, and Irelynd. Carolyn has had a baby boy, Liz's brother, Camron. I'll enjoy seeing them and telling them about their aunt Heather. As I'm sure the rest of the family will. This book is for them, as much as it is for my sanity.

In my group, when I left, one of the other widowers was asking, "how long will it take" to get over the death of his wife. I told him I would not get over it. I have learned to deal with it, and with the passage of time, it dose not hurt as bad. I still cry from time to time, but the pain is tolerable now. I'll always love her and feel her in my heart. She'll always be a part of me.

I started dating, not out of being lonely, or to try to replace what could never be replaced, but because it felt right. Was it easy? Yes. This was because it felt right. I wasn't dating to avoid being lonely. I was ready to be a single guy again. I asked the woman for a date because she intrigued me. If I wasn't going to date, it wouldn't be to the fact that I was morning my wife for the rest of my life. I didn't want to be alone because of my grief. It had been a year and nine months since Heather's death.

Her name is Deborah. She is a mother of two great kids, Rachel and Harrison. I asked her to come to a gig that the band had. She was going out of town and could not make it. The next month, she called me and we went out and had a great time, to put it politely. She even got to see the band play our last club gig that month. We've been going out for over two years now and things are going great! I've met her family, and she's met mine, Heathers' as well. I'm looking forward again, with a smile on my face. She encourages me to do the things I say, "Hey, what if?" We both have a creative side that we nurture and enjoy.

Is it the same as what Heather and I had? No. It can't be. "Deb" is a totally different lady from Heather. Although I think Heather would have liked her.

None of the women I've dated have been like the others. Everyone has different qualities, and to try and find someone who's just like the other I lost is ridiculous to me.

When I told my parents I was dating again, my mom had just the girl she thought I ought to go out with. I said thanks, but no thanks. I figured that once I started dating again, different people would want me to meet a "friend" of theirs.

Deb and I had an instant connection and I feel lucky to have met her. I didn't think I was going to fall in love again with the first woman I dated. I thought I'd do the single guy thing till I just happened upon the next girl some day, if that was even going to happen again. Wow, I didn't think it was going to happen this soon!

So that's the end of my story thus far. I hope you don't feel you wasted your time. Good luck to you and I hope the best for all of you. Take care, and remember to *be the man she loved.*

Mike